*A Gift for:*_____

From: _____

Your Psalm to Wellness

Prayers to Inspire and Motivate You to Live a Healthy & Fit Lifestyle

Your Psalm to Wellness
by Belinda Johnson
Copyright 2013 by Belinda Johnson

Publisher: EBJ Enterprises

Editor: G.E. Johnson at www.gejohnsonmedia.com

Book Interior Design: Katie Brady Design

Book Cover design: KPE Media

ISBN 978-0-615-86847-9

Dedication

To: Hubby (Eric Johnson) & Children (Chasitie and Cavonta Johnson)
Hubby, your unending love and support pushes me beyond my comfort
zone. You inspire me to live my life to the fullest. So glad I made a decision
to live and enjoy life with you. My Princess (Chat) and Prince (Cavonta)
mommy loves you both. You both are gifts from God to me!

To: Parents & Siblings
Words will never be enough to express how much I appreciate the love, sup-
port and the ways you all encourage me to go forward in life.
I love you Daddy, Mommy, Tee, Stacy, J.R. and Derrick.
Best parents and siblings a girl could ask for.

To: Spiritual Leaders
Thanks for imparting in me the Word of God that continues to catapult me
into my next wealthy place in God. Pastor Tony & Cynthia Brazelton,
Pastor Cedric & Miranda Taylor, Pastor Philip & Maricia Sherman
and Dr. Lee & Julia Ward: I thank God daily for allowing me to
have opportunities to be fed spiritual food by each of you.

To: My heaven sent friend and Sister in Christ
Maricia Sherman
All the morning manna, heart to heart talks and the tough love have shown
me that true friendship still exists. You are indeed a true friend!
As iron sharpens iron, so a friend sharpens a friend.
Proverb 27:17 NLT 2007
Love you Sis

Introduction

As I laid my head down on my pillow, so many things were on my mind that were beyond negative circumstances and it had taken a hold of me mentally, sprirtually, physically and financially. My eyes began to close and right before my eyes were shut, I saw a very, very bright light and a huge smile came on my face, it was as if a weight was lifted off of me. I immediately recognized that the Lord had entered my bedroom. I said, Yes Lord. What are you saying to me? He said, "I want you to write me a Psalm." I said hesitantly, Oh, ok. How? He answered, "I will show you. Just give me your ear and I shall speak to you and you shall write." And suddenly there it came – beautiful words in my ear that created and gave birth to Your Psalm to Wellness – a book of health and fitness prayers to help encourage, enlighten and empower you to live a healthy and fit lifestyle.

Be Motivated
Determined
Strengthened
and Inspired to B Fit

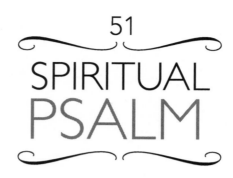

51
SPIRITUAL
PSALM

[1] Have mercy upon me, O God, according to thy lovingkindness: according unto the multitude of thy tender mercies blot out my transgressions.

[2] Wash me throughly from mine iniquity, and cleanse me from my sin.

[3] For I acknowledge my transgressions: and my sin is ever before me.

[4] Against thee, thee only, have I sinned, and done this evil in thy sight:that thou mightest be justified when thou speakest, and be clear when thou judgest.

[5] Behold, I was shapen in iniquity; and in sin did my mother conceive me.

[6] Behold, thou desirest truth in the inward parts: and in the hidden part thou shalt make me to know wisdom.

[7] Purge me with hyssop, and I shall be clean: wash me, and I shall be whiter than snow.

[8] Make me to hear joy and gladness; that the bones which thou hast broken may rejoice.

[9] Hide thy face from my sins, and blot out all mine iniquities.

[10] Create in me a clean heart, O God; and renew a right spirit within me.

[11] Cast me not away from thy presence; and take not thy holy spirit from me.

[12] Restore unto me the joy of thy salvation; and uphold me with thy free spirit.

[13] Then will I teach transgressors thy ways; and sinners shall be converted unto thee.

[14] Deliver me from bloodguiltiness, O God, thou God of my salvation: and my tongue shall sing aloud of thy righteousness.

[15] O Lord, open thou my lips; and my mouth shall shew forth thy praise.

[16] For thou desirest not sacrifice; else would I give it: thou delightest not in burn

[17] The sacrifices of God are a broken spirit: a broken and a contrite heart, O God, thou wilt not despise.

[18] Do good in thy good pleasure unto Zion: build thou the walls of Jerusalem.

[19] Then shalt thou be pleased with the sacrifices of righteousness, with burnt offering and whole burnt offering: then shall they offer bullocks upon thine altar.

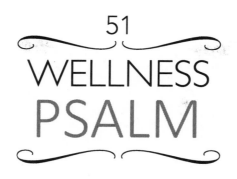

51
WELLNESS
PSALM

Fitness Starts NOW, never Later

Have mercy upon me, O God, for not taking care of my body as I should have.

Keep me away from sickness and diseases.

Wash me thoroughly from any negative thoughts or excuses when it comes to working out or eating healthy and cause me to desire to work-out and eat clean foods.

For I will confess that I've been lazy, in denial, full of excuses, out of control with my eating habits and I will take full responsibility for being out of shape.

Behold, at this point, I desire to be whole, healthy and fit in every area of my life.

Purge me from any and all things that hinder me from being effective in the kingdom of God.

I shall eat clean, workout and I shall reap the benefits of a healthy and fit lifestyle.

Make me do whatever I need to do so my bones, joints and heart will be healthy.

Create in me a healthy heart as I do my cardio daily.

Give me a right attitude toward exercising so I can be effective in the kingdom of God on earth.

Let me not go astray from what I know will keep me healthy and fit.

Deliver me from excuses, bad eating habits, negative words and laziness so I can live my best here on earth.

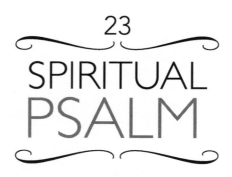

23

SPIRITUAL
PSALM

[1] The Lord is my shepherd; I shall not want.

[2] He maketh me to lie down in green pastures: he leadeth me beside the still waters.

[3] He restoreth my soul: he leadeth me in the paths of righteousness for his name's sake.

[4] Yea, though I walk through the valley of the shadow of death, I will fear no evil: for thou art with me; thy rod and thy staff they comfort me.

[5] Thou preparest a table before me in the presence of mine enemies: thou anointest my head with oil; my cup runneth over.

[6] Surely goodness and mercy shall follow me all the days of my life: and I will dwell in the house of the Lord forever.

23
WELLNESS
PSALM

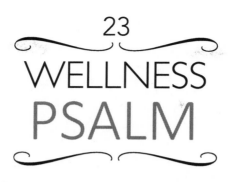

*Your fitness goals may appear to be impossible
at first, but being consistent with a plan of
Action will make it POSSIBLE*

This is my body and I shall be healthy & fit.
He giveth me the strength to exercise daily.

My body is restored, revived, renewed and rejuvenated
each time I consistently eat healthy foods.

Yea, though my flesh may be challenged, I will not fear
but I will speak and delcare over my life, good health
and strength comes to my body now! For God has
assured me with a promise that I am healed.

Surely FIT, FINE & GOOD HEALTH shall follow me all
the days of my LIFE.

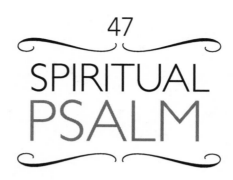

47

SPIRITUAL
PSALM

[1] O clap your hands, all ye people; shout unto God with the voice of triumph.

[2] For the Lord most high is terrible; he is a great King over all the earth.

[3] He shall subdue the people under us, and the nations under our feet.

[4] He shall choose our inheritance for us, the excellency of Jacob whom he loved. Selah.

47
WELLNESS
PSALM

Don't embrace anything that does not ADD
value, increase or profit to your life

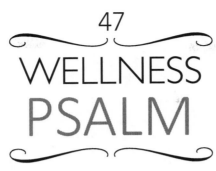

O get up and move while you can; exercise the body
God has given to you as a gift!

For the Lord most high is pleased when you do what
it takes to make yourself more effective for
the kingdom of God.

U shall stay motivated, determined, strengthened
and inspired to be fit.

God has chosen for you to live life and live it
more abundantly.

Get excited about having the strength and desire to
exercise and eat healthy.

Sing praises to God while you work out; sing praises while
you stretch your body and get involved with community
events to stay active.

Allow God to be Lord over your body.

Seek God Almighty for wisdom, ideas and directions to make
you more effective in the kingdom of God on earth.

Stay active, people of God!

Create events for the body of Christ that promote healthy
living and a fit lifestyle. God will be pleased!

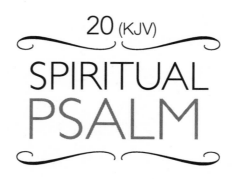

20 (KJV)
SPIRITUAL PSALM

[1] The Lord hear thee in the day of trouble; the name of the God of Jacob defend thee;

[2] Send thee help from the sanctuary, and strengthen thee out of Zion;

[3] Remember all thy offerings, and accept thy burnt sacrifice; Selah.

[4] Grant thee according to thine own heart, and fulfill all thy counsel.

[5] We will rejoice in thy salvation, and in the name of our God we will set up our banners: the Lord fulfill all thy petitions.

[6] Now know I that the Lord saveth his anointed; he will hear him from his holy heaven with the saving strength of his right hand.

[7] Some trust in chariots, and some in horses: but we will remember the name of the Lord our God.

[8] They are brought down and fallen: but we are risen, and stand upright.

[9] Save, Lord: let the king hear us when we call.

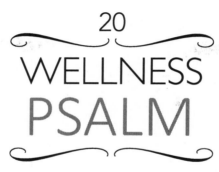

20
WELLNESS
PSALM

Be consistent with something that will improve
your quality of life

The Lord hear thee in the day when so many believers are in trouble with their health; the name El Rophe - "God our healer" - has healed us from all sickness and disease.

Lord, give us the strength to do whatever it takes to
live like Heaven on earth.

Please Daddy God do not remember our days when
we destroyed our health by making unwise
and unhealthy choices.

Grant unto us the benefits of exercising, eating healthy, resting
and drinking lots of water.

Help us accomplish living a healthy lifestyle NOW!

We will rejoice in the decision we made to live
healthy and fit.

Hear, listen and take heed, The Lord God Almighty has saved his
chosen one from an unhealthy lifestyle.

Return not to your old ways of eating and being a lazy
man full of excuses to not workout.

Let it be your RESOLVE to be consistent with this
NEW, Healthy and Fit way of living!

43 (KJV)

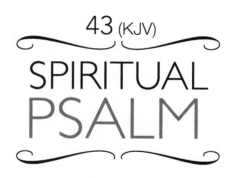

SPIRITUAL
PSALM

¹ Judge me, O God, and plead my cause against an ungodly nation: O deliver me from the deceitful and unjust man.

² For thou art the God of my strength: why dost thou cast me off? why go I mourning because of the oppression of the enemy?

³ O send out thy light and thy truth: let them lead me; let them bring me unto thy holy hill, and to thy tabernacles.

⁴ Then will I go unto the altar of God, unto God my exceeding joy: yea, upon the harp will I praise thee, O God my God.

⁵ Why art thou cast down, O my soul? and why art thou disquieted within me? hope in God: for I shall yet praise him, who is the health of my countenance, and my God.

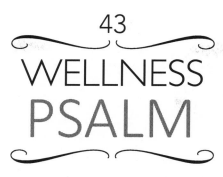

43
WELLNESS
PSALM

Invest in who or what you need to make the necessary steps toward being healthy and fit

LORD, get me out of this place of inconsistency; help me be consistent with an exercise regimen. Keep me from making excuses to not work out and eat right; help me to quit ignoring the root of the problem and burying the real issue with food as a comfort.

I counted on my own ways to cover up my hurts and disappointments; I chose to go to food as my comfort instead of coming to you as my HEALER and my own ways yielded forth bad health and an overweight body.

Why, I ask myself, am I living beneath my privileges? Why do I entertain and embrace such an unhealthy lifestyle? Enough IS Enough!

I will put my hope in God and be in good health. I will change and live a healthy and fit lifestyle. I will embrace the God of good health and fitness!

24 (KJV)

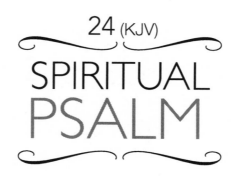

SPIRITUAL
PSALM

[1] The earth is the Lord's, and the fullness thereof; the world, and they that dwell therein.

[2] For he hath founded it upon the seas, and established it upon the floods.

[3] Who shall ascend into the hill of the Lord? Or who shall stand in his holy place?

[4] He that hath clean hands, and a pure heart; who hath not lifted up his soul unto vanity, nor sworn deceitfully.

[5] He shall receive the blessing from the Lord, and righteousness from the God of his salvation.

[6] This is the generation of them that seek him, that seek thy face, O Jacob. Selah.

[7] Lift up your heads, O ye gates; and be ye lift up, ye everlasting doors; and the King of glory shall come in.

[8] Who is this King of glory? The Lord strong and mighty, the Lord mighty in battle.

[9] Lift up your heads, O ye gates; even lift them up, ye everlasting doors; and the King of glory shall come in.

[10] Who is this King of glory? The Lord of hosts, he is the King of glory. Selah.

24
WELLNESS
PSALM

Small steps produces BIG results

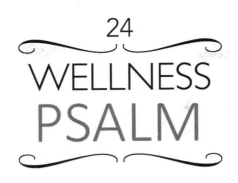

The ability to live a healthy & fit lifestyle and the potential to be successful in doing so, lies within us.

For he has given us the strength to DECIDE and it shall be established in our lives.

Who shall look and feel good in their garments? Or who shall be noticed or recognized as a person who has resolved in their heart to have a healthy,
fit and fine body?

He that has embraced life and it more abundantly, made time to prepare his meals and allows working out to be a part of his schedule and plans.

He shall receive the fruit of such action taken. Who wants to transform their mind, body & soul?

Those who apply God's word to their lives and who do their cardio and strength training consistently.

The Lord will cause them to be
FIT for his kingdom here on earth!

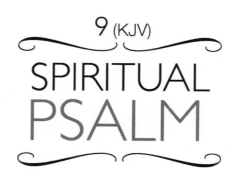

9 (KJV)

SPIRITUAL PSALM

¹ I will praise thee, O Lord, with my whole heart; I will shew forth all thy marvellous works.

² I will be glad and rejoice in thee: I will sing praise to thy name, O thou most High.

³ When mine enemies are turned back, they shall fall and perish at thy presence.

⁴ For thou hast maintained my right and my cause; thou satest in the throne judging right.

⁵ Thou hast rebuked the heathen, thou hast destroyed the wicked, thou hast put out their name for ever and ever.

⁶ O thou enemy, destructions are come to a perpetual end: and thou hast destroyed cities; their memorial is perished with them.

⁷ Arise, O Lord; let not man prevail: let the heathen be judged in thy sight.

⁸ Put them in fear, O Lord: that the nations may know themselves to be but men. Selah.

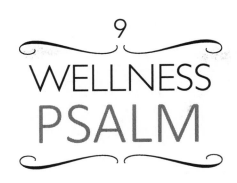

9
WELLNESS
PSALM

*Refrain from every option that will hinder
your Vision of good health*

I will lead by example, O Lord, with my decision to be healthy and fit. I will show forth results in my body with the action I have taken to live a healthy lifestyle.

I will be glad and rejoice with all of those who have resolved in their hearts to exercise and eat right.

When the enemy comes with distractions and hinderances, I will rise above his tactics with the Word of God and remain in my heavenly position, For thou hast given me the strength and the provision to maintain a healthy and fit lifestyle.

Thou hast removed and delivered me from all sicknesses, diseases, excuses and distractions that will hinder me from being fit.

O thou enemy, your plan for my life has come to a perpetual END and I have embraced LIFE and it more abundantly.

Arise, people! Let us not waste any more time becoming healthy, fit and effective for the kingdom of God on earth.

Put forth an effort to be healthy and fit. Take the opportunity while you can!

39 <small>(KJV)</small>

SPIRITUAL PSALM

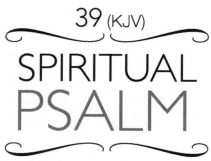

[1] I said, I will take heed to my ways, that I sin not with my tongue: I will keep my mouth with a bridle, while the wicked is before me.

[2] I was dumb with silence, I held my peace, even from good; and my sorrow was stirred.

[3] My heart was hot within me, while I was musing the fire burned: then spake I with my tongue,

[4] Lord, make me to know mine end, and the measure of my days, what it is: that I may know how frail I am.

[5] Behold, thou hast made my days as an handbreadth; and mine age is as nothing before thee: verily every man at his best state is altogether vanity. Selah.

[6] Surely every man walketh in a vain shew: surely they are disquieted in vain: he heapeth up riches, and knoweth not who shall gather them.

[7] And now, Lord, what wait I for? my hope is in thee.

[8] Deliver me from all my transgressions: make me not the reproach of the foolish.

[9] I was dumb, I opened not my mouth; because thou didst it.

[10] Remove thy stroke away from me: I am consumed by the blow of thine hand.

[11] When thou with rebukes dost correct man for iniquity, thou makest his beauty to consume away like a moth: surely every man is vanity. Selah.

[12] Hear my prayer, O Lord, and give ear unto my cry; hold not thy peace at my tears: for I am a stranger with thee, and a sojourner, as all my fathers were.

[13] O spare me, that I may recover strength, before I go hence, and be no more.

39
WELLNESS
PSALM

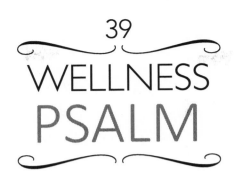

It's called a flexible meal, not a cheat meal. You can't cheat on yourself

I resolved in my heart that I will take action and do some type of exercise regimen daily. I will not allow work, school, family, church or self to get in the way of my decision to be fit.

My heart will be fixed on what I have decided and I will exercise, eat healthy and speak life over my body. I will accomplish all my health and fitness goals through Christ who strengthens me.

Lord, give me a vision to keep before me of what I will look and feel like as I press toward my fitness goals.

Behold, thou hast made me to know the truth that you desire for my life, to prosper and be in good health. Therefore, I will live in the best state that I can live in and be effective in the kingdom of God.

Hear my decree, O Lord, and give ear to my resolution, for I will do my part in order to be established as a healthy and fit child of God.

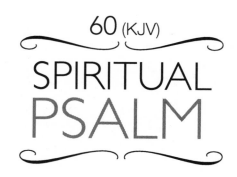

60 (KJV)

SPIRITUAL PSALM

[1] O God, thou hast cast us off, thou hast scattered us, thou hast been displeased; O turn thyself to us again.

[2] Thou hast made the earth to tremble; thou hast broken it: heal the breaches thereof; for it shaketh.

[3] Thou hast shewed thy people hard things: thou hast made us to drink the wine of astonishment.

[4] Thou hast given a banner to them that fear thee, that it may be displayed because of the truth. Selah.

[5] That thy beloved may be delivered; save with thy right hand, and hear me.

[6] God hath spoken in his holiness; I will rejoice, I will divide Shechem, and mete out the valley of Succoth.

[7] Gilead is mine, and Manasseh is mine; Ephraim also is the strength of mine head; Judah is my lawgiver;

[8] Moab is my washpot; over Edom will I cast out my shoe: Philistia, triumph thou because of me.

[9] Who will bring me into the strong city? who will lead me into Edom?

[10] Wilt not thou, O God, which hadst cast us off? and thou, O God, which didst not go out with our armies?

[11] Give us help from trouble: for vain is the help of man.

[12] Through God we shall do valiantly: for he it is that shall tread down our enemies.

60
WELLNESS
PSALM

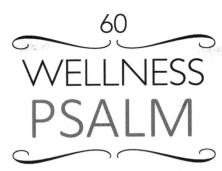

You're not frustrated enough if things haven't change because frustration gives birth to Action that produces change

Help us O God! We have ignored the many opportunities you have given us to become healthy & fit.

You have made the truth plain and clear to us that you desire for us to prosper and be in good health.

And yet, we did nothing.

Now we are out of shape, overweight, some underweight, stressed and without energy. Give us the strength to correct our foolishness and make us whole, healthy and fit.

Save us and rescue us from the control the enemy has on our mind and body. God speaks NOW and says, "I will make a way for you to live a healthy and fit lifestyle." Health is mine, says the Lord, so it belongs to you. Beauty is mine, says the Lord, so it belongs to you.

I want your PRAISE in return as I make a way for you to live a healthy and fit lifestyle.

But sickness, disease, sorry excuses, complaining and bad eating habits all belong to the devil. Keep it ALL UNDER YOUR FEET!

I allowed Jesus to nail all hinderances to the cross. Don't miss another opportunity to be healthy and fit. With you God, we will take every opportunity to exercise, make healthier food choices, live, laugh and love one another.

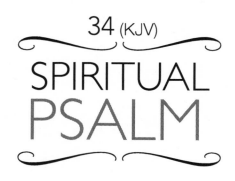

34 (KJV)

SPIRITUAL PSALM

[1] I will bless the Lord at all times: his praise shall continually be in my mouth.

[2] My soul shall make her boast in the Lord: the humble shall hear thereof, and be glad.

[3] O magnify the Lord with me, and let us exalt his name together.

[4] I sought the Lord, and he heard me, and delivered me from all my fears.

[5] They looked unto him, and were lightened: and their faces were not ashamed.

[6] This poor man cried, and the Lord heard him, and saved him out of all his troubles.

[7] The angel of the Lord encampeth round about them that fear him, and delivereth them.

[8] O taste and see that the Lord is good: blessed is the man that trusteth in him.

[9] O fear the Lord, ye his saints: for there is no want to them that fear him.

[10] He keepeth all his bones: not one of them is broken.

[11] Evil shall slay the wicked: and they that hate the righteous shall be desolate.

[12] The Lord redeemeth the soul of his servants: and none of them that trust in him shall be desolate.

34
WELLNESS
PSALM

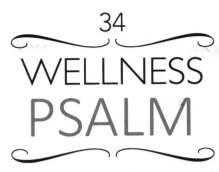

Stay committed to your Vision, not your feelings. Your feelings will have you all over in left field.

I will bless God with my body every chance I get. I live, breathe and speak God's promises that I am healthy, fit and wonderfully made.

If sickness tries to trespass, I quickly evict it with the power & authority that God has given me.

O magnify (make big the importance of) taking care of your body by exercising and eating healthy. Let us do it together as a body of believers.

I sought the Lord and he spoke. I shall live and not die and He delivered me from the fear of dying.

People looked at me with amazement and were encouraged because they saw how God healed me and made me whole, healthy and fit.

I reached out to those who were living an unhealthy lifestyle and encouraged them to change their way of living in order to add years to their lives.

O prepare your foods in healthier ways and experience the results of healthy living: Blessed is the man that chooses to live a lifestyle that includes healthy living.

Keep the body from overeating and being inactive. Depart from fattening foods and excuses to not work out!

Be consistent with your health & fitness goals, put action behind your goals, KNOW that your goals are attainable, reachable and tangible.

The Lord revives, rejuvenates and restores the body of those who honor Him with a healthy and fit lifestyle!

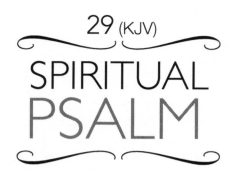

29 (KJV)
SPIRITUAL PSALM

¹ Give unto the Lord, O ye mighty, give unto the Lord glory and strength.

² Give unto the Lord the glory due unto his name; worship the Lord in the beauty of holiness.

³ The voice of the Lord is upon the waters: the God of glory thundereth: the Lord is upon many waters.

⁴ The voice of the Lord is powerful; the voice of the Lord is full of majesty.

⁵ The voice of the Lord breaketh the cedars; yea, the Lord breaketh the cedars of Lebanon.

⁶ He maketh them also to skip like a calf; Lebanon and Sirion like a young unicorn.

⁷ The voice of the Lord divideth the flames of fire.

⁸ The voice of the Lord shaketh the wilderness; the Lord shaketh the wilderness of Kadesh.

⁹ The voice of the Lord maketh the hinds to calve, and discovereth the forests: and in his temple doth every one speak of his glory.

¹⁰ The Lord sitteth upon the flood; yea, the Lord sitteth King for ever.

¹¹ The Lord will give strength unto his people; the Lord will bless his people with peace.

29
WELLNESS
PSALM

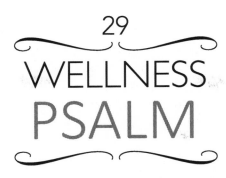

*Don't grow weary in your fitness journey. If
you keep going forward with small steps and
changes you shall reap results.*

Give unto the body what it needs on a day-to-day basis.
O ye people of God, give your best when it comes to
taking care of your temple.

Give unto the human body healthy foods and
bodily exercise.

Worship the Lord with a lifestyle of health & fitness.
The voice of the Lord speaks loud: Prosper and
be in good health.

The Lord wants us to enjoy prosperity with
a healthy body.

He created the body with the ability to skip, run, jump, walk,
swim or to have some type of movement for cardio.

The voice of the Lord speaks good health,
life and strength.

The voice of the Lord overpowers the excuses that humans
make for not exercising and not eating healthy.

The Lord has given unto us all the strength and
ability to live a healthy & fit life!

13 (KJV)

SPIRITUAL
PSALM

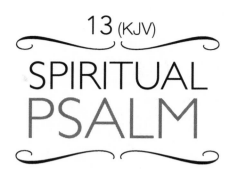

[1] How long wilt thou forget me, O Lord? For ever? how long wilt thou hide thy face from me?

[2] How long shall I take counsel in my soul, having sorrow in my heart daily? how long shall mine enemy be exalted over me?

[3] Consider and hear me, O Lord my God: lighten mine eyes, lest I sleep the sleep of death;

[4] Lest mine enemy say, I have prevailed against him; and those that trouble me rejoice when I am moved.

[5] But I have trusted in thy mercy; my heart shall rejoice in thy salvation.

[6] I will sing unto the Lord, because he hath dealt bountifully with me.

13
WELLNESS PSALM

*My family's negative health history does not
predict my future but it does help me change
my daily habits*

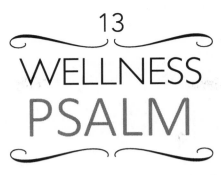

How long will you dishonor God with your body? How long will you ignore the truth - that you must take full responsibility for taking care of your body which is the temple of God?

How long shall you keep seeking or asking him for healing in your physical body and yet eat all kinds of unhealthy foods and make the excuse that you don't have time to work out?

How long will you continue to go to every healing service and put your name on the sick and shut-in list and not take ACTION to correct the bad habits that are causing so many aches, pains, sickness & disease in your body?

How long people of God? Consider!Hear!Listen! DO!

Exercise, get active, seek professional help from fitness trainers, attend health & fitness workshops to feed the mind knowledge on how to be healthy & fit and stay consistent.

In doing all of this, give God PRAISE for allowing you the opportunity to become healthy and FIT!

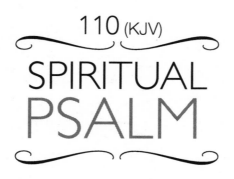

110 (KJV)
SPIRITUAL PSALM

[1] The Lord said unto my Lord, Sit thou at my right hand, until I make thine   enemies thy footstool.

[2] The Lord shall send the rod of thy strength out of Zion: rule thou in the midst of thine enemies.

[3] Thy people shall be willing in the day of thy power, in the beauties of holiness from the womb of the morning: thou hast the dew of thy youth.

[4] The Lord hath sworn, and will not repent, Thou art a priest for ever after the order of Melchizedek.

[5] The Lord at thy right hand shall strike through kings in the day of his wrath.

[6] He shall judge among the heathen, he shall fill the places with the dead bodies; he shall wound the heads over many countries.

[7] He shall drink of the brook in the way: therefore shall he lift up the head.

110

WELLNESS
PSALM

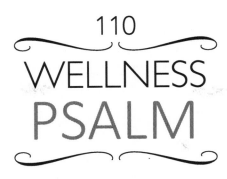

*Declutter your mind and Detox your body to
make room for your New Fit body that requires
a new way of thinking to maintain.*

The Lord said unto me, Don't just sit around all day, everyday and wait for something to happen! Get up and make something happen.

Decide, Decree and Declare what you want and watch Him establish it daily in your life.

The Lord will impart unto you ideas and instructions the moment you DECIDE and give you the strength to perform the tasks, even in the midst of your enemies saying what you will never be or what you will not accomplish.

Be willing to exercise your power and authority everyday. The Lord is true to his word; Thou art a King's child forever.

Now DROP The ROCK (the promises and word of God) on every area of your life that are not yielding increase and watch Him cause those dry places to be filled with whatever you say in Jesus name!

Exercise your God-given power to be spiritually FIT today!

3
SPIRITUAL
PSALM

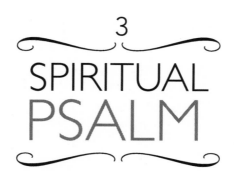

¹ Lord, how are they increased that trouble me! many are they that rise up against me.

² Many there be which say of my soul, There is no help for him in God. Selah.

³ But thou, O Lord, art a shield for me; my glory, and the lifter up of mine head.

⁴ I cried unto the Lord with my voice, and he heard me out of his holy hill. Selah.

⁵ I laid me down and slept; I awaked; for the Lord sustained me.

⁶ I will not be afraid of ten thousands of people, that have set themselves against me round about.

⁷ Arise, O Lord; save me, O my God: for thou hast smitten all mine enemies upon the cheek bone; thou hast broken the teeth of the ungodly.

⁸ Salvation belongeth unto the Lord: thy blessing is upon thy people. Selah.

3
WELLNESS
PSALM

by E. Cornell

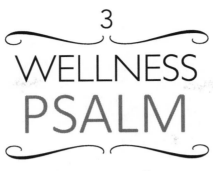

*Be careful not to return to old habits
once you've experience any amount of success
in your life*

L ord, how this weight troubles me!
Many calories - they rise up against me. Late at night,
food seems to call my soul,

But thou, O Lord, art disciplining me to take control of this
gluttony enemy.

Now the time has come for me to embrace change and live
VICTORIOUSLY!

I will not be out of control when I'm invited to a brunch or
buffet, but I will exercise my ability to have self control. I
will arise, get up and do something! For I have been given
strength to take control of my health.

Good health belongs to you; It is a blessing that
God has bestowed upon His people.

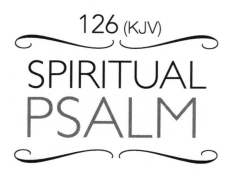

126 (KJV)

SPIRITUAL PSALM

[1] When the Lord turned again the captivity of Zion, we were like them that dream.

[2] Then was our mouth filled with laughter, and our tongue with singing: then said they among the heathen, The Lord hath done great things for them.

[3] The Lord hath done great things for us; whereof we are glad.

[4] Turn again our captivity, O Lord, as the streams in the south.

[5] They that sow in tears shall reap in joy.

[6] He that goeth forth and weepeth, bearing precious seed, shall doubtless come again with rejoicing, bringing his sheaves with him.

126
WELLNESS
PSALM

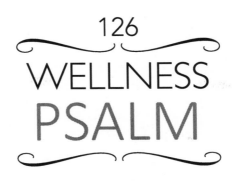

I DECLARE Life over you:
Live
Intentional
Faithfully
Everyday

When you exercise and eat right, you look good and you are full of energy. Therefore, you will fill your mouth with plenty of fresh fruits & veggies along with lean protein.

People will say, "WOW! You look GREAT!" And your response will be that the Lord has restored my health. He has turned my sickness into good health and I am reaping LIFE and it more abundantly

You will sow and invest in your health so you can enjoy all the things that He has freely given to you.

I will no longer complain about working out; I will do it with excitement, high expectations and I am looking forward to GREAT results.

127 (KJV)

SPIRITUAL PSALM

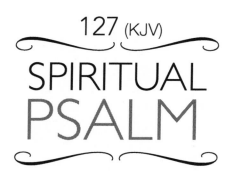

[1] Except the Lord build the house, they labour in vain that build it: except the Lord keep the city, the watchman waketh but in vain.

[2] It is vain for you to rise up early, to sit up late, to eat the bread of sorrows: for so he giveth his beloved sleep.

[3] Lo, children are an heritage of the Lord: and the fruit of the womb is his reward.

[4] As arrows are in the hand of a mighty man; so are children of the youth.

[5] Happy is the man that hath his quiver full of them: they shall not be ashamed, but they shall speak with the enemies in the gate.

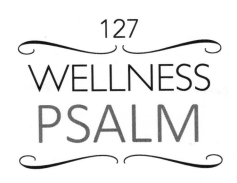

127
WELLNESS
PSALM

I AM more than a craving. I AM more than an addiction. I AM more than what he or she said I was. I AM more than a number on a scale. I AM FEARFULLY & WONDERFULLY made and so are YOU!

Except you decide in your heart to live a healthy and fit lifestyle, you will be limiting your own ability to do effective work in the kingdom.

It is vain and foolish to eat unhealthy foods and not exercise your body, then expect God's healing to flow freely in your body.

Lo, we are children of God who have been given good health and it is our job to take care of our body the temple of God.

As the power of God has been given unto us, so are we equipped to live a spiritually and physically fit life. Happy and full of joy shall those be who put effort in caring for their bodies.

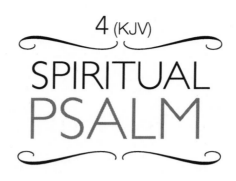

4 (KJV)

SPIRITUAL
PSALM

¹ Hear me when I call, O God of my righteousness: thou hast enlarged me when I was in distress; have mercy upon me, and hear my prayer.

² O ye sons of men, how long will ye turn my glory into shame? how long will ye love vanity, and seek after leasing? Selah.

³ But know that the Lord hath set apart him that is godly for himself: the Lord will hear when I call unto him.

⁴ Stand in awe, and sin not: commune with your own heart upon your bed, and be still. Selah.

⁵ Offer the sacrifices of righteousness, and put your trust in the Lord.

⁶ There be many that say, Who will shew us any good? Lord, lift thou up the light of thy countenance upon us.

⁷ Thou hast put gladness in my heart, more than in the time that their corn and their wine increased.

⁸ I will both lay me down in peace,and sleep:for thou, Lord,only makest me dwell in safety.

4
WELLNESS
PSALM

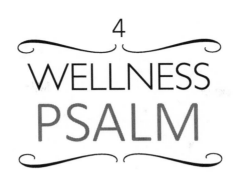

NO, NO, NO... the time is NOW!
You constantly saying later will never bring you
into your Now! Let's Go!

Hear me, O God, who desires for me to be in good health.
My body has outgrown the fearfully and wonderfully
frame you created for me to live in.

O people of God, how long will we allow stress to control how
much or how little we eat?

How long will we allow food to be our comfort? But know
that the Lord has given knowledge and wisdom to doctors,
personal trainers, group instructors and coaches to assist
you with living a healthy lifestyle. Invest in your health and
stand in amazement as the results of a healthy and fit body
are manifested!

117 (KJV)

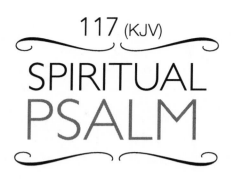

SPIRITUAL
PSALM

[1] O praise the Lord, all ye nations: praise him, all ye people.

[2] For his merciful kindness is great toward us: and the truth of the Lord endureth for ever. Praise ye the Lord.

117
WELLNESS
PSALM

Take time today and make healthy food choices intentionally!! Remember your body deserves your attention!

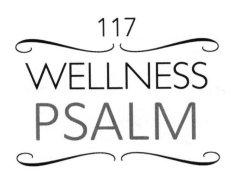

O people of the Lord all over the world, come together as a group and workout in your churches, workplace and neighborhoods.

For God's hand will be upon this outreach and so shall many lives be changed and impacted forever. Praise ye the Lord for health & fitness!

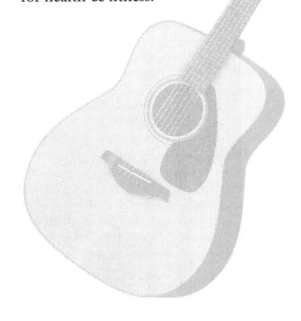

121 (KJV)

SPIRITUAL
PSALM

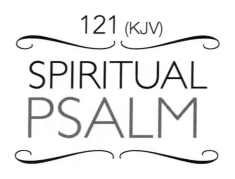

¹ I will lift up mine eyes unto the hills, from whence cometh my help.

² My help cometh from the Lord, which made heaven and earth.

³ He will not suffer thy foot to be moved: he that keepeth thee will not slumber.

⁴ Behold, he that keepeth Israel shall neither slumber nor sleep.

⁵ The Lord is thy keeper: the Lord is thy shade upon thy right hand.

⁶ The sun shall not smite thee by day, nor the moon by night.

⁷ The Lord shall preserve thee from all evil: he shall preserve thy soul.

⁸ The Lord shall preserve thy going out and thy coming in from this time forth, and even for evermore.

Psalm 121

121
WELLNESS
PSALM

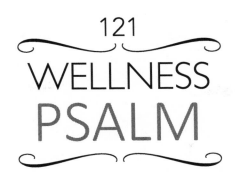

*One thing that is needed on your health and
fitness journey is an open heart for CHANGE!*

I will lift my knees as high as I can to climb these hills as I work my thighs, legs and abs.

My help cometh from the Lord who made this physical body. He will not suffer my foot to cramp as a hinderance to me working out my lower body.

The sun shall not be unbearable; therefore I will finish my workout and not use the hot weather as an excuse to give up.

The Lord shall strengthen, tone and shape my legs as I go up and down these hills.

I will stand strong and be courageous as I become healthy and FIT!

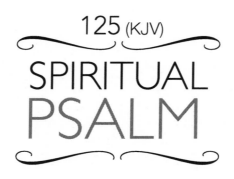

125 (KJV)

SPIRITUAL PSALM

[1] They that trust in the Lord shall be as mount Zion, which cannot be removed, but abideth for ever.

[2] As the mountains are round about Jerusalem, so the Lord is round about his people from henceforth even for ever.

[3] For the rod of the wicked shall not rest upon the lot of the righteous; lest the righteous put forth their hands unto iniquity.

[4] Do good, O Lord, unto those that be good, and to them that are upright in their hearts.

[5] As for such as turn aside unto their crooked ways, the Lord shall lead them forth with the workers of iniquity: but peace shall be upon Israel.

125

WELLNESS
PSALM

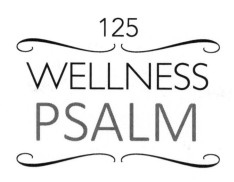

*Don't keep pushing your health to the back
burner as if you don't need a healthy & fit body
to maintain the empire you are building.*

They that workout and take in good nutrition shall reap the benefits of being healthy & fit.

As sickness & disease are all around us, so is the ever present promise of God that we are HEALED which outweighs everything else.

Therefore, we as believers will declare our healing in our body in Jesus' name.

We will eat right, exercise, drink plenty of water and get our rest and the people of God will yield forth good health and a fit body to serve effectively in the kingdom of God on earth.

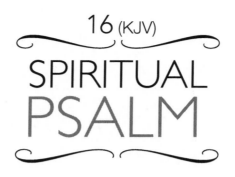

16 (KJV)

SPIRITUAL
PSALM

[1] Preserve me, O God: for in thee do I put my trust.

[2] O my soul, thou hast said unto the Lord, Thou art my Lord: my goodness extendeth not to thee;

[3] But to the saints that are in the earth, and to the excellent, in whom is all my delight.

[4] Their sorrows shall be multiplied that hasten after another god: their drink offerings of blood will I not offer, nor take up their names into my lips.

[5] The Lord is the portion of mine inheritance and of my cup: thou maintainest my lot.

[6] The lines are fallen unto me in pleasant places; yea, I have a goodly heritage.

[7] I will bless the Lord, who hath given me counsel: my reins also instruct me in the night seasons.

[8] I have set the Lord always before me: because he is at my right hand, I shall not be moved.

[9] Therefore my heart is glad, and my glory rejoiceth: my flesh also shall rest in hope.

[10] For thou wilt not leave my soul in hell; neither wilt thou suffer thine Holy One to see corruption.

[11] Thou wilt shew me the path of life: in thy presence is fulness of joy; at thy right hand there are pleasures for evermore.

16
WELLNESS
PSALM

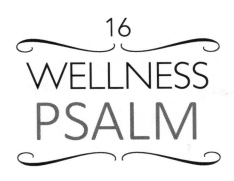

*Are you HEARING what your body is telling
you it needs? Take heed and listen. Become
aware and recognize what is needed to take you
to a healthier place!*

Preserve me, O God, for I put my life in your hands.
  O, my heart and body will I give to you.

I will keep before me a vision of what I want my body to look like and make time for a daily workout routine; I shall not be distracted.

Therefore my heart will be healthy, my body will be full of energy and my flesh shall rest well at night. For thou will give me the strength to stay steady and faithful in living a healthy lifestyle.

Thou wilt show me the pathway of healthy living and in following your instructions is a lifestyle of being fit, fine, fabulous and healthy forevermore.

113 (KJV)

SPIRITUAL
PSALM

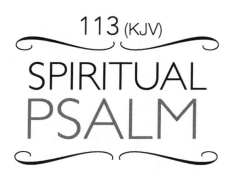

¹ Praise ye the Lord. Praise, O ye servants of the Lord, praise the name of the Lord.

² Blessed be the name of the Lord from this time forth and for evermore.

³ From the rising of the sun unto the going down of the same the Lord's name is to be praised.

⁴ The Lord is high above all nations, and his glory above the heavens.

⁵ Who is like unto the Lord our God, who dwelleth on high,

⁶ Who humbleth himself to behold the things that are in heaven, and in the earth!

⁷ He raiseth up the poor out of the dust, and lifteth the needy out of the dunghill;

⁸ That he may set him with princes, even with the princes of his people.

⁹ He maketh the barren woman to keep house, and to be a joyful mother of children. Praise ye the Lord.

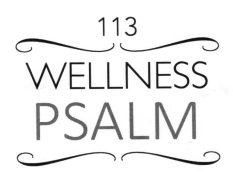

113
WELLNESS
PSALM

*You Are Healthy & FIT, not because of a shape
or size but because it is a Promise of God!*

Praise ye the Lord for the potential and the ability to make my life more enjoyable!

O ye servants of the Lord, you have the strength of God to exercise and eat healthy.

Blessed be the name of the Lord from the time I strike out with my morning run until I lay my head down for good sleep.

From day to day shall I offer God a healthy and fit body because I choose to live in good health.

The Lord keeps my spirit lifted as I work toward achieving my weight loss goals.

Who is willing to take control of their health?

You are says the LORD!

He raiseth up the tired and overworked bodies and places His strength inside them to workout and cook healthy meals, so that they may teach others how to be healthy & fit.

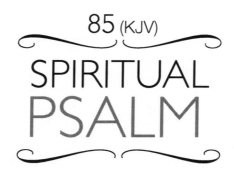

85 (KJV)

SPIRITUAL PSALM

[1] Lord, thou hast been favourable unto thy land: thou hast brought back the captivity of Jacob.

[2] Thou hast forgiven the iniquity of thy people, thou hast covered all their sin. Selah.

[3] Thou hast taken away all thy wrath: thou hast turned thyself from the fierceness of thine anger.

[4] Turn us, O God of our salvation, and cause thine anger toward us to cease.

[5] Wilt thou be angry with us for ever? wilt thou draw out thine anger to all generations?

[6] Wilt thou not revive us again: that thy people may rejoice in thee?

[7] Shew us thy mercy, O Lord, and grant us thy salvation.

[8] I will hear what God the Lord will speak: for he will speak peace unto his people, and to his saints: but let them not turn again to folly.

[9] Surely his salvation is nigh them that fear him; that glory may dwell in our land.

[10] Mercy and truth are met together; righteousness and peace have kissed each other.

[11] Truth shall spring out of the earth; and righteousness shall look down from heaven.

[12] Yea, the Lord shall give that which is good; and our land shall yield her increase.

[13] Righteousness shall go before him; and shall set us in the way of his steps.

85
WELLNESS
PSALM

Embrace the truth & take Action to
preserve your health!

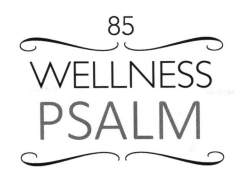

Lord, thou hast healed my body, thou hast restored my health.

Thou hast forgiven me for mistreating my body.

Thou hast renewed my mind when it comes to my health.

Help me, O God, to trust you for complete healing and cause all manner of diseases that tries to attack me to cease.

Thank you God for allowing your son Jesus to put to death all sickness & disease at the cross. Thank you for making my body effective for the kingdom of God on earth. For my ears are open to hear your instructions daily on how to take care of my body.

For you will speak to me what, when, where and how to build and maintain a healthy & fit mind, body and soul and I will not only hear but I will be a doer of your instructions.

But let me not turn again to my old bad eating habits and lazy attitude toward exercising.

Yea, the Lord shall give me a tone, healthy and fit body.

My body shall show forth the fruit of a person who is determined, dedicated and disciplined to be fit!

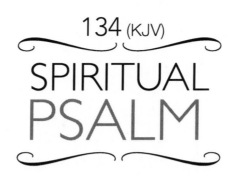

134 (KJV)

SPIRITUAL
PSALM

[1]Behold, bless ye the Lord, all ye servants of the Lord, which by night stand in the house of the Lord.

[2] Lift up your hands in the sanctuary, and bless the Lord.

[3] The Lord that made heaven and earth bless thee out of Zion.

134
WELLNESS
PSALM

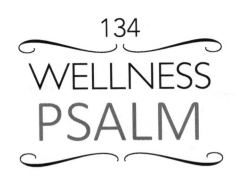

*Honor your body today by making a Decision
to take care of the vehicle that takes you
everywhere you have to go!*

Behold! Check this out, servants of the Lord! Give attention to your body; feed it lean protein, good whole grains as carbs and good fats every day. Workout your body consistently and worship the

Father with your lifestyle.

The Lord who made heaven and earth will bless your effort in taking care of your body.

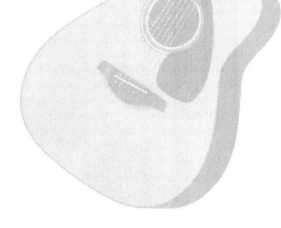

138 (KJV)

SPIRITUAL PSALM

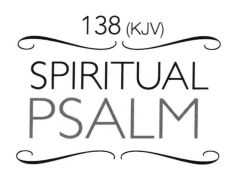

¹I will praise thee with my whole heart: before the gods will I sing praise unto thee.

²I will worship toward thy holy temple, and praise thy name for thy lovingkindness and for thy truth: for thou hast magnified thy word above all thy name.

³In the day when I cried thou answeredst me, and strengthenedst me with strength in my soul.

⁴All the kings of the earth shall praise thee, O Lord, when they hear the words of thy mouth.

⁵Yea, they shall sing in the ways of the Lord: for great is the glory of the Lord.

⁶Though the Lord be high, yet hath he respect unto the lowly: but the proud he knoweth afar off.

⁷Though I walk in the midst of trouble, thou wilt revive me: thou shalt stretch forth thine hand against the wrath of mine enemies, and thy right hand shall save me.

⁸The Lord will perfect that which concerneth me: thy mercy, O Lord, endureth for ever: forsake not the works of thine own hands.

138
WELLNESS
PSALM

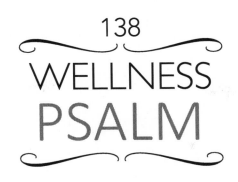

*Never follow your negative feelings about
exercising because when those feelings are gone;
you are left without Results.*

I will praise thee as I run my miles, swim my laps or ride my bike.

I will become determined, disciplined in my mind
and dedicated to offering my body to you as the temple of God.

On the days that my flesh tries to make me choose fried foods
instead of baked foods or cakes and cookies over fresh fruit,
I will remind myself that you are God, my source and my strength.

All the people in the body of Christ shall be excited about
working out and eating healthy.

Yea, we shall find ways and time to stay healthy and fit.

No longer as brothers and sisters will we allow one another to
do harmful things to our body. But we will encourage one
another to do things that promote health and wellness.

The Lord will perfect that hindrance that gets in the way of us
being healthy and fit.

71 (KJV)

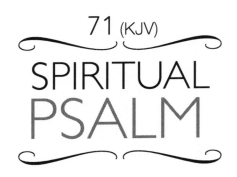

SPIRITUAL PSALM

¹ In thee, O Lord, do I put my trust: let me never be put to confusion.

² Deliver me in thy righteousness, and cause me to escape: incline thine ear unto me, and save me.

³ Be thou my strong habitation, whereunto I may continually resort: thou hast given commandment to save me; for thou art my rock and my fortress.

⁴ Deliver me, O my God, out of the hand of the wicked, out of the hand of the unrighteous and cruel man.

⁵ For thou art my hope, O Lord God: thou art my trust from my youth.

⁶ By thee have I been holden up from the womb: thou art he that took me out of my mother's bowels: my praise shall be continually of thee.

⁷ I am as a wonder unto many; but thou art my strong refuge.

⁸ Let my mouth be filled with thy praise and with thy honour all the day.

⁹ Cast me not off in the time of old age; forsake me not when my strength faileth.

¹⁰ For mine enemies speak against me; and they that lay wait for my soul take counsel together,

¹¹ Saying, God hath forsaken him: persecute and take him; for there is none to deliver him.

¹² O God, be not far from me: O my God, make haste for my help.

¹³ Let them be confounded and consumed that are adversaries to my soul; let them be covered with reproach and dishonour that seek my hurt.

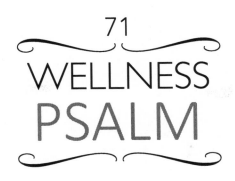

71
WELLNESS
PSALM

*I DIVORCED my unhealthy habits; they
became too much of a burden for me to carry.*

In thee do I put my life in your hands Lord.
Let me never live beneath my privileges again.

Deliver me into good health and cause me to escape bad
health. Keep me Focus and consistent with healthy living.
Be thou my strength when it is time to workout, whereunto
I may continue to exercise.

Deliver me O my God from eating chocolate all month,
skipping meals and unhealthy desires. Let my mouth be
filled with healthy balance meals daily and with the right
amount of water each day.

Let me not fall into a "I'm getting too old and can't do this
Attitude" but give me the strength to continue the journey
of living healthy & fit.

My body shall have tone arms, legs and abs all the days
of my life, for my heart will perform the way God designed
it, For I will not be ashame of my body
because I choose to be FIT!

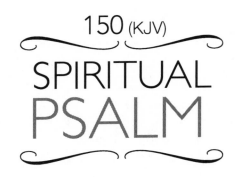

150 (KJV)

SPIRITUAL
PSALM

[1]Praise ye the Lord. Praise God in his sanctuary: praise him in the firmament of his power.

[2] Praise him for his mighty acts: praise him according to his excellent greatness.

[3] Praise him with the sound of the trumpet: praise him with the psaltery and harp.

[4] Praise him with the timbrel and dance: praise him with stringed instruments and organs.

[5] Praise him upon the loud cymbals: praise him upon the high sounding cymbals.

[6] Let every thing that hath breath praise the Lord. Praise ye the Lord.

150
WELLNESS
PSALM

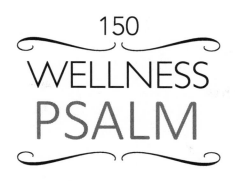

*Don't become a carrier of things that weigh
you down, that can cause more than a number
on a scale to go up*

Praise Ye the Lord for a healthy & fit body. Praise Him for strength to exercise. Praise Him for the ability to eliminate aches & pains by working out your body.

Praise Him for blood that circulates properly throughout your body.

Praise Him for a lifestyle change. Praise Him for a healthy heart.

Praise Him for an excellent immune system.

Praise Him for the strength and ability to do what it takes to keep your body in tip top shape!

Let all who are able and without EXCUSES; exercise, eat healthy, drink plenty of water and get plenty of rest.

15 (KJV)

SPIRITUAL PSALM

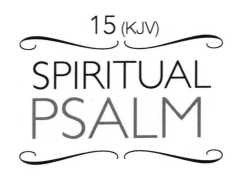

¹ Lord, who shall abide in thy tabernacle? Who shall dwell in thy holy hill?

² He that walketh uprightly, and worketh righteousness, and speaketh the truth in his heart.

³ He that backbiteth not with his tongue, nor doeth evil to his neighbour, nor taketh up a reproach against his neighbour.

⁴ In whose eyes a vile person is contemned; but he honoureth them that fear the Lord. He that sweareth to his own hurt, and changeth not.

⁵ He that putteth not out his money to usury, nor taketh reward against the innocent. He that doeth these things shall never be moved.

15
WELLNESS
PSALM

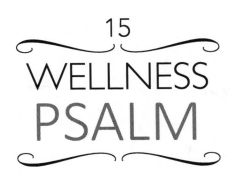

You got to learn not to listen to anything that
goes against your fitness regimen.

Lord, who can live healthy and fit? Who shall look young and be active in their old age?

He that exercises consistently, puts clean and healthy foods inside his body, and gets proper rest; He that does not overeat at buffets or parties, nor sits and watches the exercise dvd, nor gets upset when told that he needs to do something about his health.

But he that stays focused and on course with a fitness plan, cuts out all stress and drama and understands the importance and value of taking care of the body - he shall live healthy and fit all the days of his life.

133 (KJV)

SPIRITUAL PSALM

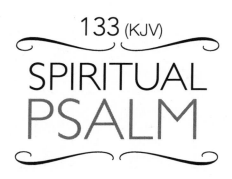

¹Behold, how good and how pleasant it is for brethren to dwell together in unity!

² It is like the precious ointment upon the head, that ran down upon the beard, even Aaron's beard: that went down to the skirts of his garments;

³ As the dew of Hermon, and as the dew that descended upon the mountains of Zion: for there the Lord commanded the blessing, even life for evermore.

133
WELLNESS
PSALM

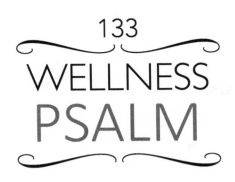

I heard, I listened, I conquered...I SMILE!
Don't be afraid to challenge yourself.

Behold, how exciting and fruitful it is when the members of the body of Christ take charge of their health! It is so awesome when pastors and leaders can flow in the anointing and teach their flock how to be spiritually and physically fit.

As they take the lead by being consistent with applying the word of God to their lives, exercising and choosing to eat clean; then shall they see the fruit of a spiritually and physically fit church.

112 (KJV)

SPIRITUAL PSALM

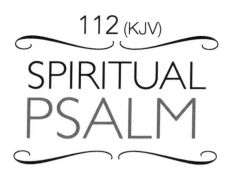

¹Praise ye the Lord. Blessed is the man that feareth the Lord, that delighteth greatly in his commandments.

² His seed shall be mighty upon earth: the generation of the upright shall be blessed.

³ Wealth and riches shall be in his house: and his righteousness endureth for ever.

⁴ Unto the upright there ariseth light in the darkness: he is gracious, and full of compassion, and righteous.

⁵ A good man sheweth favour, and lendeth: he will guide his affairs with discretion.

⁶ Surely he shall not be moved for ever: the righteous shall be in everlasting remembrance.

⁷ He shall not be afraid of evil tidings: his heart is fixed, trusting in the Lord.

⁸ His heart is established, he shall not be afraid, until he see his desire upon his enemies.

⁹ He hath dispersed, he hath given to the poor; his righteousness endureth for ever; his horn shall be exalted with honour.

¹⁰ The wicked shall see it, and be grieved; he shall gnash with his teeth, and melt away: the desire of the wicked shall perish.

112
WELLNESS
PSALM

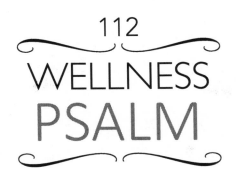

Listen to instructions.
Process now but a SMILE Later!

Praise ye the Lord! I have finally started doing what it takes to have a healthy & fit lifestyle.

I shall lead by example for my family to follow.

My family shall be blessed as we take steps toward our health & fitness goals.

Wealth, health and fitness shall be a part of our lifestyle and our endurance to run, walk, swim or jog shall last at least 30 minutes a day.

Unto us creative ideas shall come to us on how to get our community involved in becoming fit for the Kingdom of God on earth.

Surely we will not give in to chocolate, chips, cake or candy, but we will remember to practice self-control.

We will not be afraid of losing our motivation to exercise and to eat right. Our heart is fixed on being a healthy and fit sister, brother, mother, father, son or daughter.

We have given our money to gyms that we never attended and made resolutions that we did not keep, but our efforts will become ACTION that yields forth results because we are not just talking the talk, but walking it OUT!

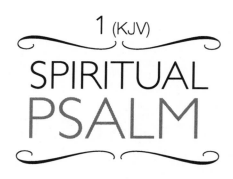

1 (KJV)

SPIRITUAL PSALM

[1] Blessed is the man that walketh not in the counsel of the ungodly, nor standeth in the way of sinners, nor sitteth in the seat of the scornful.

[2] But his delight is in the law of the Lord; and in his law doth he meditate day and night.

[3] And he shall be like a tree planted by the rivers of water, that bringeth forth his fruit in his season; his leaf also shall not wither; and whatsoever he doeth shall prosper.

[4] The ungodly are not so: but are like the chaff which the wind driveth away.

[5] Therefore the ungodly shall not stand in the judgment, nor sinners in the congregation of the righteous.

[6] For the Lord knoweth the way of the righteous: but the way of the ungodly shall perish.

1
WELLNESS
PSALM

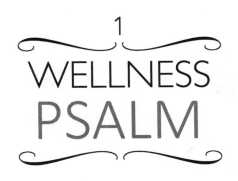

Fitness is like music to my body.
Sing body Sing!

Blessed is the man that does not become a couch potato, nor a lazy man full of excuses, nor a person that does excessive eating and drinking.

But he shall be like a man full of action, power and purpose; He plans his meals and works his plan.

He allows edifying music to assist him as he walks, runs or jumps for cardio and he shall not allow anything or anyone get in the way of him lifting up the name of Jesus as he lifts those weights for strength training.

For the Lord knows what it takes to keep him motivated, determined, strengthened and inspired to be FIT!

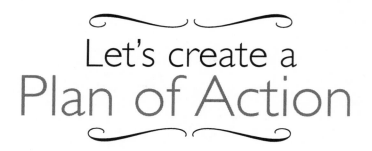

Let's create a
Plan of Action

1. What fitness ACTION can you APPLY to your life daily?

_____

_____

_____

_____

_____

_____

2. How can you CHANGE your eating habits?

_____

_____

_____

_____

_____

_____

3. How can you TEACH others the importance of taking care of their body?

_____

_____

_____

_____

_____

_____

4. Create a daily health and fitness affirmation to SAY everyday!

_____

_____

_____

_____

_____

If you have enjoyed this book, Coach "B" Fit
would love to hear from you.

Please send comments to
info@IamCoachBFIT.com

Thank you!